Persuasive Foods

To

Lose Weight

And

Live Vigorously

by

Dr. Scott D. Nauman

TABLE OF CONTENTS

TABLE OF CONTENTS..3

INTRODUCTION 4

Chapter 1 8

Fat Burning fundamentals 8

Chapter 2 12

Fat smoldering Foods 12

Chapter 3 21

Persuasive Foods 21

INTRODUCTION

You are not a bad person if you are overweight. Simply overweight, you are. However, losing weight is essential for improving your appearance, improving your health, and boosting your sense of self-worth. You will need to maintain your weight after losing the fat.

You will learn how to lose 10 pounds in a month, or about two or two-and-a-half pounds per week, safely and painlessly in this book. You won't feel deprived, and you'll be happier and more active than you were before.

The majority of Americans gain weight by consuming unhealthy foods. The key to success over the long term is changing these bad eating habits. The key is both the right food and knowledge.

When people lived in caves, they had no idea how to preserve and store food. They hunted and gathered food with all of their waking energy. They devoured it quickly once they had it. They burned fat for energy during times when there was little or no food available, rather than storing food in cupboards or pantries.

During the hot sprints and summer months, they needed to put on a substantial amount of fat each year. That was the only way they could ensure that they would survive the cold, harsh winter months.

Additionally, since women bear children, they typically weigh more because they require more energy to support themselves and their offspring.

Even though we no longer live in caves, our hunter-gatherer ancestors left us with this fundamental mechanism for fat storage.

There are a certain number of fat cells in each person at birth. Your genetic makeup determines how many of these fat cells you have. If you have a lot of fat cells, it's possible that your ancestors were the biggest people in the tribe, which was good because it meant that they were more likely to live.

Fat cells can never be removed, but you can unfortunately add to them. Your body will make new far cells based on what you eat. And they never go away, just like the ones you were born with.

That does not mean that once you gain weight, you will always be fat. Fat cells can be reduced in size. When you lose weight, you experience that. The fat that is stored in those large fat cells is burned off. They're like balloons. The same effect as releasing air from a balloon is achieved by burning the fat that is contained within them.

A certain amount of calorie restriction is necessary for a successful weight loss program. You lose weight by eating less fat and exercising more.

You need to change the kinds of foods you eat to reduce your intake of fat while still getting the vitamins, minerals, trace elements, protein, fat, and carbohydrates your body needs to thrive to guarantee a lifetime of weight control success.

Diets with a lot of calories may help you lose weight quickly, but in the long run, they won't work.

This is because humans have a genetic resistance to starvation. Our bodies slow down their metabolisms and burn less energy to keep us alive when there isn't enough food.

By establishing a "set point," the hypothalamus, a region of the brain, maintains an even weight. That is the weight at which we are most at ease. Based on the level of consumption it is accustomed to, the hypothalamus determines this point. Even if that point is higher than it ought to be, it aims to maintain our constant weight.

The brain thinks the body is starving when we drastically reduce our food intake, so it slows the metabolism to keep life going. Soon, the weight loss stops. As a result, we eat more as we feel full and uncomfortable. The diet then fails.

How can you make up for the slowdown in your metabolism? The solution is to alter the nutritional content of the foods you consume. To lose weight, you must reduce your total calorie intake, which is essential. However, reducing the number of calories you consume from fat is more important.

That's how you won't experience panic or starvation in your system. You also reduce the amount of fat in your food by substituting safe, low-calorie, nutrient-dense plant foods for it. Your brain will be persuaded by this that your body is getting everything it needs from food.

You will be able to consume fewer calories and fats while eating more food and feeling fuller longer.

Plant foods are high in vitamins, minerals, trace elements, carbohydrates, and protein for energy and muscle building, and they break down slowly in your stomach to give you a longer feeling of fullness. Your body can burn off the excess fat it has stored thanks to this.

Chapter 1
Fat Burning fundamentals

You are not a bad person if you are overweight. Simply overweight, you are. However, losing weight is essential for improving your appearance, improving your health, and boosting your sense of self-worth. You will need to maintain your weight after losing the fat.

You will learn how to lose 10 pounds in a month, or about two or two-and-a-half pounds per week, safely and painlessly in this book. You won't feel deprived, and you'll be happier and more active than you were before.

The majority of Americans gain weight by consuming unhealthy foods. The key to success over the long term is changing these bad eating habits. The key is both the right food and knowledge.

When people lived in caves, they had no idea how to preserve and store food. They hunted and gathered food with all of their waking energy. They devoured it quickly once they had it. They burned fat for energy during times when there was little or no food available, rather than storing food in cupboards or pantries.

During the hot sprints and summer months, they needed to put on a substantial amount of fat each year. That was the only way they could ensure that they would survive the cold, harsh winter months.

Additionally, since women bear children, they typically weigh more because they require more energy to support themselves and their offspring.

Even though we no longer live in caves, our hunter-gatherer ancestors left us with this fundamental mechanism for fat storage.

There are a certain number of fat cells in each person at birth. Your genetic makeup determines how many of these fat cells you have. If you have a lot of fat cells, it's possible that your ancestors were the biggest people in the tribe, which was good because it meant that they were more likely to live.

Fat cells can never be removed, but you can unfortunately add to them. Your body will make new far cells based on what you eat. And they never go away, just like the ones you were born with.

That does not mean that once you gain weight, you will always be fat. Contracting fat cells is conceivable. When you lose weight, you experience that. The fat that is stored in those large fat cells is burned off. They're like balloons.

The same effect as releasing air from a balloon is achieved by burning the fat that is contained within them.

A certain amount of calorie restriction is necessary for a successful weight loss program. You lose weight by eating less fat and exercising more.

You need to change the kinds of foods you eat to reduce your intake of fat while still getting the vitamins, minerals, trace elements, protein, fat, and carbohydrates your body needs to thrive to guarantee a lifetime of weight control success.

Diets with a lot of calories may help you lose weight quickly, but in the long run, they won't work.

This is because humans have a genetic resistance to starvation. Our bodies slow down their metabolisms and burn less energy to keep us alive when there isn't enough food.

By establishing a "set point," the hypothalamus, a region of the brain, maintains an even weight. That is the weight at which we are most at ease. Based on the level of consumption it is accustomed to, the hypothalamus determines this point. Even if that point is higher than it ought to be, it aims to maintain our constant weight.

The brain thinks the body is starving when we drastically reduce our food intake, so it slows the metabolism to keep life going. Soon, the weight loss stops. Thus, we become ravenous and awkward and afterward eat more. The diet then fails.

How can you make up for the slowdown in your metabolism? The solution is to alter the nutritional content of the foods you consume. To lose weight, you must reduce your total calorie intake, which is essential. However, reducing the number of calories you consume from fat is more important.

That's how you won't experience panic or starvation in your system. You also reduce the amount of fat in your food by substituting safe, low-calorie, nutrient-dense plant foods for it. Your brain will be persuaded by this that your body is getting everything it needs from food.

You will be able to consume fewer calories and fats while eating more food and feeling fuller longer.

Plant foods are high in vitamins, minerals, trace elements, carbohydrates, and protein for energy and muscle building, and they break down slowly in your stomach to give you a longer feeling of fullness. Your body can burn off the excess fat it has stored thanks to this.

Chapter 2

Fat smoldering Foods

Clinical studies have shown that the following foods help people lose weight. These foods do more than just give you no fat in your system; they also have special properties that give your system more zip and help your body lose weight. These amazing foods can curb your cravings for junk food and provide your body with clean fuel and effective energy to keep it running smoothly.

These foods can be included in any sensible weight loss plan. They provide your body with the additional metabolic boost it needs to quickly lose weight.

There should be no less than 1,200 calories per day in a healthy weight loss plan. However, if you believe Dr. Charles Klein, you should consume between 1,500 and 1,800 calories per day. He claims that even at that intake level, you will still be able to lose weight without putting your health at risk.

By filling the stomach, hunger is satisfied more completely. The following foods do that better than any other ounce-for-ounce. They also have special fat-melting abilities and are high in nutrients.

Apples

These wonders of nature merit their standing for fending the specialist off when you eat one per day. Additionally, it now appears that they can assist you in losing weight.

First of all, they last longer than most foods and raise blood glucose (sugar) levels safely and gently. According to researchers, this has the practical effect of keeping you satisfied for longer.

Second, they are one of the supermarkets' richest sources of soluble fiber. According to Dr. James Anderson of the University of Kentucky's School of Medicine, this kind of fiber guards against dangerous swings or drops in your blood sugar level, preventing hunger pangs.

A medium-sized apple contains no sodium, saturated fat, or cholesterol and only 81 calories. By lowering your blood pressure and lowering the amount of cholesterol already present in your body, you will also reap additional health benefits.

Whole-Grain Bread

No need to be afraid of bread. The bread itself is not fattening; rather, what you put on it—cream cheese, butter, or margarine—is. We'll repeat it as often as necessary: fat makes you fat. Consider this: a gram of carbohydrate has four calories, a gram of protein has four, and a gram of fat has nine. If that doesn't convince you, consider this: So which of these makes you fat?

Bread is safe for dieting because it is a natural source of complex carbohydrates and fiber. Dr. Bjarne Jacobsen, a Norwegian scientist, discovered that people who consume fewer than two slices of bread per day weigh approximately 11 pounds more than those who consume a lot of bread.

Learns at Michigan State College show a few slices of bread diminish hunger. White bread and dark, high-fiber bread were compared, and it was found that students who consumed 12 slices of dark, high-fiber bread daily felt less hungry and lost five pounds in two months. Others who consumed white bread experienced increased hunger consumed more fatty foods, and did not lose any weight.

Consuming dark, dense, and high-fiber loaves of bread like pumpernickel, whole wheat, mixed grain, oatmeal, and others are therefore essential. Whole grain bread has surprising amounts of protein and only 60 to 70 calories per slice. It is also high in complex carbohydrates, which are the best, most stable fuel for your body.

Coffee

Easy is the key here and it works. Caffeine has been linked to several negative effects, including insomnia and anxiety, and moderation is the key.

Coffee's caffeine has the potential to accelerate metabolism. According to Dr. Judith Stern of the University of California at Davis, it is referred to as a metabolic enhancer in nutritional circles.

Given that caffeine is a stimulant, this makes sense. Concentrates on how it can assist you with consuming a bigger number of calories than typical, maybe up to 10 percent more. It is best to drink one cup in the morning and one cup in the afternoon for your safety. Try it without sugar and only use skim milk; many people come to love it that way.

Grapefruit

This traditional diet food should be a regular part of your diet for good reason. Dr. James Cerd of the University of Florida asserts that it aids in the dissolution of cholesterol and fat. A grapefruit of average size has 74 calories, 15 grams of pectin (a special fiber that helps lower cholesterol and fat), a lot of vitamin C and potassium, and no fat or sodium.

It has a lot of natural galacturonic acid, which makes it better at fighting fat and cholesterol. This also aids in the fight against atherosclerosis, which is the hardening of the arteries, and the onset of heart disease. To lessen the tart flavor, sprinkle it with cinnamon rather than sugar.

Mustard

Try the spicy, hot kind from Asian import shops, specialty stores, and exotic grocery stores. Like caffeine and the drug ephedrine, Dr. Jaya Henry of Oxford Polytechnic Institute in England discovered that the amount of hot mustard typically used in Mexican, Indian, and Asian recipes—roughly one teaspoon—temporarily speeds up metabolism. Henry responds, "But mustard is completely natural and safe."It is effective and can be used every day. It can accelerate metabolism by as much as 20% to 25% for several hours, which surprised me. According to Dr. Henry, this can cause the body to burn an additional 45 calories for every 700 calories consumed.

Peppers

Henry asserts that hot, spicy chili peppers are comparable to hot mustard. He tested them under the same conditions as the mustard and discovered that they functioned similarly. A meal with 766 calories totals contained only three grams of chili peppers. Henry refers to this as a "diet-induced thermic effect" because the peppers' metabolism-boosting properties worked like a charm. The effect is easily achieved with little effort. There are only four to eight chilies in the majority of salsa recipes.

Peppers have just 24 calories per cup, are low in sodium, contain a lot of calcium, phosphorus, iron, magnesium, and vitamins A and C, and are high in fiber.

Potatoes

We can't be serious, can we? Wrong. It's unfair that potatoes get the same bad rap for being "fattening" as bread." An excellent food with which to achieve rapid weight loss is the potato, at 0.6 calories per gram or approximately 85 calories per potato," states Dr. John McDougal, director of the nutritional medicine clinic at St. Helena Hospital in Deer Park, California. They lower cholesterol and protect against stroke and heart disease. They are also a great source of potassium and fiber.

Toppings and preparation are crucial. You will fail if you include butter, milk, and sour cream. Instead, opt for yogurt.

Rice

Dr. William Kempner, a researcher at Duke University in Durham, North Carolina, came up with the Rice Diet, a comprehensive weight loss plan that is easy to understand. Rice is a staple of the diet, which dates back to the 1930s. You gradually incorporate a variety of fruits and vegetables later.

It has remarkable weight loss and medical benefits. It has been demonstrated that diet can reverse kidney disease and lower blood pressure.

A cup of cooked rice (150 grams) contains around 178 calories - roughly 33% of the number of calories tracked down in an identical measure of hamburger or cheddar. Also, keep in mind that whole-grain rice is much healthier than white rice.

Soups

Drinking soup is healthy! Old-fashioned, homemade soup is better for weight loss than canned versions from the store. According to a study conducted by Dr. John Foreyt of Baylor College of Medicine in Houston, Texas, dieters who consumed soup before lunch and dinner lost more weight than those who did not. They lost more weight the more soup they ate. Additionally, soup eaters typically lose weight more quickly.

Naturally, the soup you consume has an impact. Cream soups and beef or pork soups are not your best options. However, here is a great recipe:

Slice three large onions, three carrots, four celery stalks, one yellow squash, and one zucchini.In a kettle, place.

Three cans of crushed tomatoes, two packets of low-sodium chicken bouillon, three cans of water, and one cup of white wine (if desired) should be added. Thyme, basil, oregano, tarragon, and garlic powder should be added. After boiling, simmer for an hour. Serves six.

Spinach

According to Dr. Richard Shekelle, an epidemiologist at the University of Texas, Spinach Popeye knew what he was talking about. Spinach can speed up the metabolism, reduce cholesterol, and burn fat. It provides the majority of the nutrients you require and is high in iron, beta-carotene, and vitamins C and E.

Tofu

You can't say enough good things about this Asian health food. It's also known as soybean curd. Because it doesn't taste much, you can add any flavor or spice you want to it. A 21/2-inch square contains nine grams of protein and 86 calories. A daily intake of about 40 grams is recommended by experts.)Tofu has iron and calcium, almost no sodium, and no saturated fat. It also lowers cholesterol and speeds up your metabolism. The firmer tofu can be stir-fried or added to soups and sauces, while the softer tofu can be mashed, chopped, and added to salads. There are various varieties.

Chapter 3
Persuasive Foods

Even if a few foods are delicious, nutritious, and filling, it would be unrealistic to think that you could successfully lose weight and enjoy what you eat. As a result, in addition to the excellent foods mentioned in the previous section, we are going to include a further list of fat-fighting foods.

They provide a wide range of vitamins, minerals, proteins, and other essential nutrients, as well as a variety of flavors and textures that can be incorporated into any meal. Naturally, each one has high fiber content, low-fat content, and safe sodium content.

Many have the flavor and crunchiness we've come to expect from snack foods. If you are like the majority of us, you may have a real habit of snacking on junk food, which you will need to change if you want to lose weight. A lot of the foods in this section might be good alternatives.

Barley

This satiating grain performs better than rice and potatoes. It has a respectable amount of protein and fiber per cooked cup, 170 calories, and relatively little fat. Roman gladiators complained when they had to eat meat because they needed strength from this grain.

Barley, according to research conducted at the University of Wisconsin, has potent anti-cancer properties and effectively lowers cholesterol by up to 15%. It can also help people lose weight and treat constipation better than laxatives, according to Israeli scientists.

It can be added to stews and soups as an alternative to rice in salads, pilaf, and stuffing. For a unique texture, you can also combine it with rice. When ground into flour, it makes delicious muffins and bread.

Beans

One of the best sources of plant protein is beans. The legume family includes chickpeas, beans, and peas. The majority of common beans, including lima beans, have 215 calories per cup when cooked. They are high in potassium but low in sodium, and have the least amount of fat and the most protein of any food.

Since plant protein is not complete, you must add something to make it complete. To provide the amino acids necessary to create a complete protein, combine beans with a whole grain like rice, barley, wheat, or corn. Then, with only a small amount of fat, you get the same high-quality protein as meat.

Regular consumption of beans has been shown to lower cholesterol levels in studies conducted in the Netherlands and at the University of Kentucky.

Beans are most frequently criticized for causing gas. The U.S. Department of Agriculture (USDA) suggests limiting that issue as follows: Remove any foreign particles from the beans before cooking by rinsing them and putting them in a kettle covered with boiling water. Let them soak for at least four hours, then remove any beans that float to the top and cook them in fresh water.

Berries

This is the ideal food for losing weight. Berries contain sufficient fiber to reduce calorie absorption and satisfy your sweet tooth thanks to their natural fructose sugar. British researchers discovered that fruits, vegetables, and whole grains' high content of insoluble fiber reduce calorie absorption sufficiently to promote weight loss without compromising nutrition.

Berries are a good source of potassium, which can help you control your blood pressure. Blueberries have 81 calories per cup, raspberries 60 calories per cup, and strawberries 45 calories per cup. So, have fun with the berry of your choice and use your imagination.

Broccoli

According to a recent survey, broccoli is the most popular vegetable in the United States. Why not? Only 44 calories are contained in a cup of cooked broccoli. It is regarded as the most effective cancer-fighting vegetable and provides a staggering nutritional value. It contains no fat, a lot of fiber, indoles—chemicals that fight cancer—carotene, 21 times the recommended daily allowance of vitamin C, and calcium.

Take note of the broccoli's color when you buy it. The minuscule florets ought to be deep green without any yellowing. Stems ought to be sturdy.

Buckwheat

Buckwheat is delicious in pancakes, pieces of bread, cereal, soups, and a grain dish known as kasha on its own. Each cooked cup contains 155 calories. Buckwheat-based diets, according to the All India Institute of Medical Sciences, improve blood sugar regulation, prevent diabetes, and lower cholesterol levels. Buckwheat is prepared similarly to rice and barley. Add the grain, cover the pan, reduce the heat, and simmer for 20 minutes, or until the water is absorbed, in two to three cups of water.

Cobbage

The staple of Eastern Europe, cabbage, is truly a wonder food. A cup of cooked shredded cabbage has only 33 calories, and no matter how long you cook it, all of its nutrients remain intact. It is sufficient to prevent colon cancer to consume cabbage raw (18 calories per cup of shredded cabbage), cooked, as sauerkraut (27 calories per cup of drained cabbage), or as coleslaw (calories vary depending on the dressing) once per week. Additionally, it may be a food that improves longevity. According to surveys conducted in Japan, Greece, and the United States, those who consume a lot of it have the lowest rates of death and colon cancer overall.

Carrots

What list of healthy and fat-burning foods would be complete without the favorite of Bugs Bunny? A medium-sized carrot conveys around 55 calories and is a healthful force to be reckoned with. Beta carotene, also known as provitamin A, is the powerful antioxidant that gives this food its orange hue.

Grate them into rice, chop them and toss them with pasta, or add them to a stir-fry. For flavorful dishes, combine them with parsnips, oranges, raisins, lemon juice, chicken, potatoes, broccoli, or lamb. Add tarragon, dill, cinnamon, or nutmeg to flavor them. Chopped carrots add a natural sweetness to soups and spaghetti sauce without the need for sugar.

Chicken

White chicken has 245 calories per four-ounce serving, while dark chicken has 285. Zinc, niacin, protein, and iron are all abundant in them. The healthiest kind of chicken is skinned, but most experts say to wait until the meat is done cooking to remove the skin because it keeps the meat moist.

Corn

Corn, which is a grain and not a vegetable, is another food that has received bad press. It is false to believe that it has little nutritional value. One cup of cooked kernels has 178 calories. It is high in potassium, iron, and zinc, and researchers at the University of Nebraska claim that it also provides high-quality protein.

The Tarahumara Indians of Mexico only consume beans and corn. According to Virgil Brown, M.D., of Mount Sinai School of Medicine in New York, cardiovascular heart disease and high blood cholesterol are almost nonexistent among them.

Cottage Cheese we had to include cottage cheese because we're talking about foods that help burn fat and lose weight. In addition to providing respectable amounts of calcium and the B vitamin riboflavin, low-fat (2%) cottage cheese has 205 calories per cup and is admirably low in fat. For more flavors, add herbs like dill or garden-fresh vegetables like scallions and chives.

Add raisins or one of the unsweetened fruit spreads to make it sweeter. Cottage cheese can also be used in cooking, baking, fillings, and dips where sour cream or cream cheese would normally be used.

Figs

Fiber-rich figs have only 37 calories per medium raw fig (2.25 inches in diameter) and 48 calories per dried fig.

According to a recent USDA study, they prevent overeating and contribute to a feeling of fullness. When subjects were fed a diet with more figs than a diet with the same number of calories, they complained that they were being asked to overeat.

Serve them with cheese and other fruits. Alternatively, you can cook them in fruit juice and serve them hot or cold. They can be filled with mild white cheese or pureed for use in low-calorie pastries and cookies.

Fish

Experts have always regarded fish as a healthy food because of its numerous health benefits.

The average four-ounce serving of deep-sea fish contains 236 calories, ranging from 90 calories for abalone to 236 calories for herring. For instance, water-packed tuna has 154 calories. Consuming seafood makes it hard to gain weight.

Articles published in the New England Journal of Medicine in 1985 demonstrated a clear link between regular fish consumption and lower heart disease rates.

The reason is that fish oils thin the blood, lower cholesterol, and lower blood pressure.

At Albany Medical College in New York, Dr. Joel Kremer discovered that taking fish oil supplements daily significantly reduced the inflammation and stiffness of rheumatoid arthritis joints.

Greens

Greens include turnip, mustard, Swiss chard, collard, chicory, beet, and kale. One of the super-stars, spinach, is in the same family as all of them. A cup of plain cooked greens cannot contain more than 50 calories, no matter how hard you try.

They are fat-free, high in fiber, and packed with vitamins A and C. They can be used in salads, soups, casseroles, and other dishes where spinach would normally be used.

Kiwi

With only 46 calories per fruit, Kiwi is a sweet treat from New Zealand. Officials in charge of public health in China commend the tasty fruit for its abundance of potassium and vitamin C. It keeps for up to a month in the refrigerator easily. The fuzzy skin is edible, but most people prefer it peeled.

Leeks

These giant scallions of the onion family are just as nutritious and delicious as their more well-known relatives. With just 32 calories per cooked cup, they come close to being calorie-free.

You can marinate halved leeks in vinaigrette or season them with Romano cheese, fine mustard, or herbs after poaching or broiling them. They are also excellent in soup.

Lettuce

Despite widespread belief to the contrary, lettuce is extremely nutritious. At 10 calories per cup of raw romaine, you can't leave it out of your diet plans. It packs a lot of bulk and is low in calories. Additionally, it is high in vitamin C. To spice up your salads, try Boston, bibb, and cos lettuce, as well as watercress, arugula, radicchio, dandelion greens, purslane, and even parsley.

Melons

Now, here a low-calorie option with great flavor and nutrition! There are 62 calories in a cup of cantaloupe balls, 44 calories in a cup of casaba balls, 62 calories in a cup of honeydew balls, and 49 calories in a cup of watermelon balls. They are delicious and contain some of the highest amounts of fiber of any food. A healthy food that is unrivaled in its ability to burn fat is made possible by the substantial amounts of vitamins A and C and a whopping 547 milligrams of potassium contained in that cup of cantaloupe.

Oats

Oat bran or oatmeal has 110 calories in a cup. Oats also aid in weight loss. In Dr. James Anderson's landmark 12-year study at the University of Kentucky, subjects simply consumed 100 grams (3.5 ounces) of oat bran daily and lost three pounds in two months. Just don't expect oats to do miracles on their own; for total health, you need to eat a well-balanced diet.

Onions

Onions should be a regular part of your diet because they are flavorful, fragrant, inexpensive, and low in calories. There are only 42 calories in a raw medium onion of 2.15 inches in diameter and 60 calories in a cup of chopped raw onions.

They may be useful in preventing allergic reactions, thinning the blood, controlling cholesterol, and protecting against cholesterol. Most importantly, onions are good for you and taste good.

Bake after being partially boiled, peeled and brushed with olive oil and lemon juice. Or you can spread them on pizza after sautéing them in white wine and basil. Alternately, roast them in sherry and serve them with paste.

Pasta

From the beginning, the Italians were correct. A cup of cooked paste without a thick sauce has only 155 calories and is a great staple that focuses on starches. According to research conducted by the American Institute of Baking, pasta contains manganese, iron, phosphorus, copper, magnesium, and zinc. Whole-wheat pasta, which is even healthier, should also be taken into consideration.

Sweet Potatoes

You won't feel hungry after eating sweet potatoes, and you can make a meal out of them without worrying about gaining a pound. There are about 103 calories in a sweet potato. One of the best things you can eat for vitamin A is creamy orange flesh.

They are microwaveable, steamed, or baked. or include them in a variety of casseroles, soups, and other dishes. Flavor with vegetable broth or lemon juice in place of butter.

Tomatoes

A 2.5-inch-diameter medium tomato only contains about 25 calories. These delights from the garden are low in sodium and fat, packed with potassium, and high in fiber.

According to a survey conducted at Harvard Medical School, people who consume tomatoes (or strawberries) every week have the lowest risk of dying from cancer.

Additionally, stewed, whole, peeled, and canned tomatoes should not be overlooked. They retain their nutritional value and low-calorie status while enhancing the flavor of sauces, casseroles, and soups. When served over pasta, even plain old spaghetti sauce burns fat, so consider including tomatoes in your diet.

Turkey

Give thanks to the pilgrims who started the wonderful tradition of Thanksgiving turkey. It just so happens that this meat-like health food is good all year long for losing weight.

White meat turkey has 177 calories per four-ounce serving, while dark meat has 211.

Sadly, many people are still unaware of ground turkey's versatility and flavor. Ground turkey is capable of performing at least as well as hamburgers, including conventional burgers, spaghetti sauce, and meatloaf.

The skin on some ground turkey slightly raises the fat content. Ground breast meat is best if you want to keep it very lean.

However, because this contains no additional fat, you will need to add filler to keep meatloaf or burgers together.

The amount of fat and calories in four ounces of ground turkey is roughly equivalent to 2.5 teaspoons of butter or margarine. Amazingly, the same amount of regular ground beef (21 percent fat) contains 23 grams of fat and 298 calories.

Purchasing turkey is now simple. Buying a whole bird is no longer necessary unless you want to. Drumsticks, thighs, breasts, and cutlets, as well as individual parts of the turkey, are available fresh or frozen.

Yogurt

The low-fat and non-fat varieties of plain yogurt each contain 144 calories per cup. Like all dairy foods, it has a lot of protein, is high in calcium, and it has zinc and riboflavin.

Yogurt can be used as a breakfast food by cutting up a banana and adding your favorite cereal to it.

It can be used in sauces, soups, dips, toppings, stuffings, and spreads, among other cooking applications. A straightforward funnel for making yogurt cheese is even available from many departments of kitchen gadgets.

In many dishes, yogurt can be used in place of heavy cream and whole milk, saving a lot of calories and fat.

You can substitute some or all of the ingredients with more fat. Be original. Instead of adding fat-laden sour cream to a baked potato, use yogurt, garlic powder, lemon juice, a pinch of pepper, and Worcestershire sauce instead.

There are a variety of yogurts available at health food stores and supermarkets, many of which contain sugar and fruit added. Purchase plain, non-fat yogurt and add fruit yourself to control calories and fat content. An excellent method for transforming plain yogurt into a delectable sweet treat is to use apple butter or fruit spreads that contain little or no added sugar.